W9-BZJ-835

Quit Smoking

Stop Smoking Now
Quickly And Easily
The Best All Natural And Modern
Methods To Quit Smoking

By Ace McCloud
Copyright © 2013

Disclaimer

The information provided in this book is designed to provide helpful information on the subjects discussed. This book is not meant to be used, nor should it be used, to diagnose or treat any medical condition. For diagnosis or treatment of any medical problem, consult your own physician. The publisher and author are not responsible for any specific health or allergy needs that may require medical supervision and are not liable for any damages or negative consequences from any treatment, action, application or preparation, to any person reading or following the information in this book. Any references included are provided for informational purposes only. Readers should be aware that any websites or links listed in this book may change.

Table of Contents

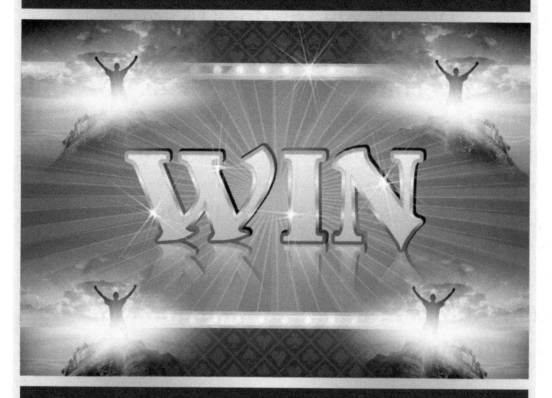

DEDICATED TO THOSE WHO ARE PLAYING THE GAME OF LIFE TO WIN

KEEP ON PUSHING AND NEVER GIVE UP!

Ace McCloud

Be sure to check out my website for all my Books and Audio books.

www.AcesEbooks.com

Introduction

I want to thank you and congratulate you for buying the book, *Quit Smoking Now, Quickly and Easily*

This book contains proven steps and strategies on how to quit smoking effectively and for the long-term. All the methods discussed in this book have been used by real people who have successfully broken their smoking addiction and habit.

It's important to remember that not every method will work for everyone, however this book offers a wide variety of hints, tips, and strategies so that you can find what works best for you.

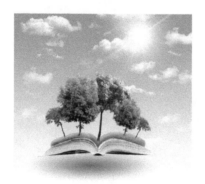

Chapter 1: What Smoking does to you

It's important to remember just how much damage smoking does to you. Sometimes, it may feel like you don't care, you just have to have that cigarette. While many smokers like the taste, and the feelings of relaxation and well-being that smoking tobacco can give you, it is actually doing quite the opposite. The lethal chemicals contained in tobacco are causing a whole chain reaction of dangerous biological events throughout every part of your body. While you may feel relaxed, your body is going through hell.

Chemicals in Cigarettes

Cigarette smoke not only contains tar, which is a solid, sticky compound of chemicals that sticks to the inside of your lungs, it also contains a lethal mixture of other chemicals such as acrolein, nitrosamines, polycyclic hydrocarbons, butadiene, chromium, polonium, formaldehyde, cadmium, benzene, arsenic, hydrogen cyanide, carbon monoxide, nitrogen oxide and ammonia. And that's not a complete list. These chemicals are used in a variety of industries including rubber manufacturing, nuclear applications, and preserving corpses. Acrolein has even been used as a chemical weapon.

What these Chemicals do to you

Just about everybody knows that smoking can cause lung cancer. That fact has been made in the media, and by governments, health officials, and anti-smoking charities. As if the risk of lung cancer wasn't enough, ninety percent of all lung cancer deaths are attributed to smoking. And lung cancer isn't the only type of cancer that smoking causes; mouth cancer, gum cancer, and throat cancer are all attributed to smoking.

It isn't only your lungs that are at risk: Your heart is at risk as well! A variety of cardiovascular diseases outnumber smoking related lung cancer deaths every year. Smoking can cause your arteries to become narrow, and when that happens, clots can form. These clots can cause thrombosis in the brain, causing a stroke, or in the heart, causing a heart attack. If the clots travel to your kidneys, then they can cause kidney failure and high blood pressure, and if they travel to your legs, they can cause gangrene. Left long enough, gangrenous limbs can require amputation.

Chapter 2: Preparing to Quit Smoking

Quitting smoking is one of the most important steps you can take towards leading a happier, healthier life. While many people wake up one morning and decide to go 'cold turkey', these people are seldom successful long-term and soon find themselves back in the habit again. With quitting smoking, preparation is everything and increases the chances of your efforts being successful exponentially.

Benefits and Motivation

If you've decided to quit smoking, which if you've bought this book, chances are good that you have, well done. That's the biggest step to make, and knowing your reasons why you're quitting smoking will stand you in good stead during the quitting process.

Besides the very real chance of a slow and painful death through emphysema, lung cancer, or heart disease, now is a good time to think about the other reasons why you should quit smoking. Have a read through this list, and think about each point in turn. If it sounds like a good reason to you, then list it in a diary or notepad for easy reference. You can refer back to this list anytime you may start to doubt yourself or your motivations for quitting smoking.

- Improved health.

- You don't have to keep going outside in the freezing cold or rain or the baking hot sun every time you want a smoke. You won't have to stop the car and get out for a smoke if you have passengers in your vehicle. You'll be able to watch a movie all the way through without having to leave the cinema or living room so you can have a quick smoke.

- You won't have to kiss and hug your children or significant other stinking of cigarette smoke – just because you can't smell it, doesn't mean that they can't.

- Whiter teeth and a brighter smile. Yellowing of the teeth is caused by tar buildup. After quitting, you will be able to brush away this tar and begin the process of restoring the natural whiteness of your teeth.

- Food will taste a lot nicer as your taste buds repair themselves – and imagine all the delicious meals you can go out for with all the money you're saving by not smoking.

- Breathing more easily. No more rattling breaths and no more squeaking and wheezing. Imagine being able to get to the top of a flight of stairs without having to stop and catch your breath.

- No more stained fingers. Those yellow stains between your fingers are caused by tar – the same substance that is sticking to the inside of your lungs. This will come off eventually after you have quit smoking completely.

- A better sex life. Imagine how great it's going to be when you don't feel like you have an ashtray in your mouth when you settle down with your partner for a sexy smooch. And don't forget, smoking impedes blood flow to your sexual organs, which can cause a lackluster performance, deadened feelings, lack of desire, and, in some cases, total impotence. Forget taking sexual enhancements medications: quit smoking. You'll be very happy with the results.

- Lots more money to spend. If you're sick of going to the store and having to go without things that you really want, but always find the money for a pack of cigarettes, let this bit of mathematics do the talking. Take the price of a pack of your favorite brand of cigarettes and divide that by twenty. That's the cost per cigarette. Now, multiply the cost per cigarette by how many cigarettes you smoke per day. This is the daily savings you'll make by quitting. Write that down. Multiply that by seven. That's your weekly savings. Write that down. Multiply that figure by four and a third. That's your monthly savings. Write that down. Finally, multiply that figure by twelve. That's your yearly savings. Write that down.

- If those numbers aren't incentive enough for you to quit smoking, try cutting some pictures out of a magazine of items that you would really love to buy but can't afford because your spending so much money on cigarettes and stick them into your notepad. You'll be amazed at the things you'll be able to afford to buy after you've quit.

Obviously, this is not a complete list of the benefits, as there are many more, so take some time to think and write down any other reasons that are personal to you and your family.

Triggers

Now it's time to think about why you smoke and when you smoke. First let's look at why you smoke. Why did you start smoking? Was it to make yourself look cool in front of your high school friends? Did you start smoking to get accepted as part of a group? Was smoking a big part of your family life when you were growing up? Whatever your reasons were for lighting up that first cigarette, now is the time to admit them to yourself and write it down in your diary or notepad.

Now let's look at why you smoke. For example, many smokers use smoking as a way of managing stress; they go outside and have a smoke and some 'fresh' air.

This gives the smoker a break from a stressful environment, and allows them to feel the 'rush' that smokers find addictive. Or, do you like to light up after a heavy meal? Do you enjoy smoking while you're talking on the phone? Do you find that you only smoke when you're drinking in a bar? Or does coffee seem lackluster without a cigarette to accompany it?

Try keeping a diary for a week. Note down the times you went for a cigarette and what you were doing immediately before going for the cigarette. Also note how you were feeling before your cigarette and how you feel after your cigarette. After a week, try to identify any patterns or triggers to your smoking habit. This will help you when your quit date arrives.

Picking your Quit Smoking Date

This may seem easy. Surely any day will do, right? If you think that, you couldn't be further from the truth. When you select a date to quit, make sure it is the least stressful day you can possibly have. Don't allow yourself to be bored, with absolutely nothing to do, just make sure you won't be doing anything on that day that is highly stressful, or that you know you will have to participate in things that trigger your smoking habit. For example, if you like a smoke when you drink alcohol, make sure you don't pick the date of your office party to quit on.

Building a Support Network

While going through the quitting process, you may feel the need to talk to someone about the way you're feeling and the side effects that you may be having. Sleeplessness, constipation, and anxiety are all common side effects of quitting smoking. It may be helpful to choose a person or people whom have quit smoking themselves because they'll be able to empathize with you and give you encouragement. They may also have some great ideas to help you cope that you may not have considered before.

Knowing your Body is Getting Healthier

The benefits of quitting smoking begin within twenty minutes. After this time, your heart rate and blood pressure will have returned to normal, and your blood circulation will improve.

After eight hours, your blood oxygen levels will have returned to that of a non-smoker, and your chances of suffering a heart attack falls significantly.

After twenty-four hours, all carbon monoxide will have left your bloodstream, and your lungs will start to get rid of tar, debris, and mucus.

After forty-eight hours, all nicotine will be out of your system, and your senses of smell and taste will have improved as taste buds recover.

After seventy-two hours, your breathing will have drastically improved. Try climbing a flight of stairs and see for yourself. Also, you will notice your libido improving and that you have considerably more energy. Now's a good time to go for a long walk and enjoy the feeling of fresh air filling your lungs instead of a toxic cocktail of lethal chemicals.

Between two and twelve weeks, circulation throughout your entire body will have improved. You'll notice that getting around is easier and takes less effort.

Between three and nine months your body will have gone through a lot of changes. Your lung efficiency will have improved by up to ten percent, and breathing problems as a result of smoking will be at a minimum if not gone entirely. Any coughing or wheezing you used to experience will have become a thing of the past.

After five years, the chances of you suffering a heart attack will have fallen to half of that of a smoker, and after ten years, your chances will be the same as someone who has never smoked in their lives. Also, your risk of lung cancer will now be half of that of a smoker.

While it's impossible to return your body to the exact state it was in before you smoked your first cigarettes, it's important to remember that the changes your body will go through as a result of quitting smoking are hugely significant in living a better, healthier life; changes that may well save your life.

Don't Diet and Quit Smoking at the Same Time

You've already got enough to deal with when you quit smoking. By adding the stress of adhering to a new dietary regimen in your life, you are drastically lowering your chances of quitting smoking successfully. Most doctors and scientists will tell you the same thing: Quit first, and worry about your diet later. Smoking does far more damage to your body than putting on a few extra pounds.

Keeping yourself Busy

During the quitting smoking process, your mind may often turn to thoughts of smoking. Many ex-smokers have mentioned that thinking about cigarettes is like thinking about an old friend, but they acknowledge that smoking is anything but your friend. So to keep these thoughts to a minimum, it is important to remember to keep yourself busy, but don't get involved in anything too stressful. Long-lasting distractions work best. Try reading a novel all in one go, or have a movie marathon. You'll be surprised at how little you think about that 'old friend' while you're doing something that you really enjoy.

Break the Habit

Don't forget that smoking is not only an addiction, it's a habit. So, it's important to try and break any old routines during which you reach for a cigarette. If you like a cigarette with your coffee after breakfast, drink some orange juice instead and then do something else fun and productive. If you like a cigarette after your favorite TV show, record the TV show and go for a walk instead. Watch the show at a different time of the day, and go do the dishes after the show. The list of routine changes you can make is endless, but it's important that they're made so you can break the habit of smoking as well as the nicotine addiction. If you would like some help with this, then I would highly recommend my book: Influence, Willpower, and Discipline.

Chapter 3: Time Tested Methods To Quit Smoking

There is no guaranteed method to ensure that you will quit smoking successfully. However, being successful often requires you to manage the side effects of the quitting smoking process. Sometimes, people relapse into a smoking habit again because they don't like the side effects of quitting. It's important to remember that these side effects are only temporary, and some people don't suffer any of them at all. Managing the side effects of the quitting process effectively is one of the most important factors to consider during the process.

Manage the Side Effects of Quitting

Nicotine cravings are typically at their worst during the first week of your quit smoking plan, but they can keep hitting you for a long time after. The best strategies will be personal to you, but many ex-smokers have reported that taking a brisk walk is highly effective in getting past a craving. Another good idea is to distract yourself. Try listening to your favorite song and singing along at full blast. Don't be embarrassed, and do whatever it takes. Another good strategy reported by ex-smokers was to simply wait it out. The more you face up to the craving – and win – the more willpower you develop and that typically reduces the occurrence of future cravings and reduces the amount of time it takes for future cravings to pass.

The irritability and impatience that can accompany nicotine withdrawals tend to disappear after two to four weeks. Ex-smokers reported that caffeine consumption made them more irritable and suggested that avoiding drinks containing caffeine helped manage this side effect. You can also take a hot bath as a relaxation technique, or do any sort of exercise to increase endorphin levels.

A big problem for many people trying to quit smoking is insomnia, which lasts about the same time as irritability symptoms – about two to four weeks. Again, the avoidance of caffeine was suggested by ex-smokers, particularly after six in the evening. A good amount of daily exercise was also cited as a good method of making sure you're tired enough to fall asleep naturally. You could also use relaxation techniques prior to going to bed, such as reading, having a warm caffeine-free drink such as milk or sleepy time tea, and a few melatonin capsules.

Typically as a result of insomnia, fatigue is a common problem for people who are trying to quit smoking. This will usually last as long as the irritability and insomnia lasts, around 2-4 weeks. It is important not to push yourself too hard during this time, and, if insomnia is not a particular issue for you, you could try taking a nap during the day if time allows.

Lack of concentration affects some people more than others during the quitting process and is typically short-lived, only lasting a week or two. It's important to try and reduce your workload during this time and avoid as much stress as possible. Some meditation may be of use here, as well as incorporating some relaxation techniques into your daily routine.

Ex-smokers often report hunger as a side effect of quitting smoking. This is caused by your metabolism returning to normal and food tasting better as your taste buds begin the restoration process. To avoid too much weight gain as a result of your increased appetite, try to eat healthier snacks such as fruit instead of candy, and reduced-calorie drinks instead of their full-calorie counterparts. After several weeks, this side effect will subside and you can start concentrating on shedding any extra weight you may have gained during this time. Smoking is doing a lot more damage to your body than carrying around a few extra pounds for a couple of weeks. Keep that in mind.

As your lungs begin to get rid of the tar, debris, and mucus that may be causing you breathing difficulties, you may experience coughing, a dry throat, or a nasal drip for a few weeks. Use cough drops to help manage coughing, but it is important not to suppress your cough entirely. Coughing is your body's way of getting rid of all that unhealthy buildup in your lungs.

Drinking plenty of fluids is the best option for controlling dry throat and coughing symptoms.

Another common side effect of those who are trying to quit smoking is constipation and associated gas. This should only last a week or two as your metabolism returns to normal along with your digestive function. During this time, ex-smokers reported that increasing your fiber intake was an excellent way of relieving these symptoms, as was drinking plenty of fluids. A daily walk was also reported to be helpful. For a more detailed look at easy ways to overcome constipation, you can check out my book: Constipation Cure.

Chapter 4: All-natural Ways to Quit Smoking

There is a whole range of products that you can buy to help with your smoking cessation efforts. Sometimes, people don't want to use more nicotine to help them get over their existing nicotine addiction. Instead, they prefer to use an all-natural way instead. Many of these methods may require a bit more willpower than using a nicotine replacement therapy like a patch or gum, but many people feel that this is the best way to quit: facing up to your addiction and dealing with it head on. This doesn't work for everyone, but if you're looking for a more natural way to quit smoking, this section is for you.

Change what you eat

There have been several recent studies performed that suggest that changing your diet increases your chances of quitting smoking successfully. The results boil down to this: Some foods make cigarettes taste better than others. By replacing the foods in your diet that make cigarettes taste good with foods that make them taste bad, your brain will begin to divert itself from 'wanting' a cigarette'. One example of this is to replace your favorite 'pre-cigarette' snack or drink with an apple or glass of apple juice. Try it. You'll be amazed at how foul cigarette smoke tastes after eating an apple or drinking apple juice.

Exercise

Performing a little bit of exercise every day can help to reduce the urge to smoke. It doesn't have to be a ten mile run to be effective, either. Recent studies have shown that a brisk walk of about a mile every day helps to curb cravings. By releasing endorphins into your body, and increasing your heart rate, your brain replaces the craving for nicotine with one for endorphins. Also, exercise will help clear all the tar and chemicals from your lungs. When you start breathing clean air, you'll soon decide cigarettes just aren't worth it.

Find a Group

Try to find a local group of other people who are quitting smoking or have quit. Sharing experiences is a great way to deal with the changes you're going through as a result of smoking cessation. If you don't like going to meet ups, try finding an internet based group. There are plenty of them out there. You could even try Twitter. Friends and Family are also a great source of inspiration and I think many of them would support you in your decision to quit and help you in any way they can.

Visual aversion

Use the internet to find images of tumors, damaged lungs, birth defects, and gangrene that have been caused by the chemicals contained in cigarette smoke.

The next time you don't think you can handle your cravings, take a look at these images and imagine that's what is happening to your own body. The craving will most likely quickly disappear.

Chapter 5: Modern Methods To Quit Smoking

Since the dangers of smoking were made public, many companies were formed with the objective of providing products that would help people to quit smoking successfully. Some of the products discussed below have been around for longer than others, but just because it has a longer history does not necessarily mean that it's right for you. As always, it's best to discuss the various smoking cessation products available with your healthcare provider or pharmacist so that you can choose the right product for you that will give you the best possible chances to quit smoking successfully.

Nicotine Gum

If you will miss the oral aspects of smoking, nicotine gum might be a good nicotine replacement tool for you to use. When you have a craving, you chew the gum and then tuck it into the corner of your mouth between your tongue and gum line. Nicotine is absorbed through the skin and helps you get in control of your cravings.

Nicotine Patches

Nicotine patches are also a very good method of nicotine replacement. You simply apply the patch to your skin and it delivers a steady slow release of nicotine into your bloodstream and helps to curb your cravings. There are many varieties and strengths available, and so it is a good idea to speak to your pharmacist or healthcare professional to decide which one to use. If you tend to wake up in the night craving for a cigarette, using a sixteen hour or twenty four hour patch is advisable, as these continue to work while you're asleep.

Nicotine Inhalator

Some ex-smokers report that they miss the action of smoking. A nicotine inhalator looks a lot like a cigarette and you have to perform the 'hand to mouth' action of smoking to get the nicotine delivered into your system. However, critics of this method suggest that you are simply replacing one addiction for another.

Nicotine Microtabs

Some people report unpleasant tastes in their mouth when using nicotine gums. If this applies to you, perhaps Microtabs are the solution you're looking for. All you need to do is place the microtab on the surface or underneath of your tongue and allow it to dissolve. As with nicotine gum, the nicotine is delivered through your skin.

Nicotine Lozenges

Nicotine lozenges can be sucked for up to thirty minutes. Nicotine delivery is through the skin and the digestive system. Lozenges come in a variety of flavors, and any unpleasant tastes are masked by flavorings such as mint or orange. This method releases the nicotine more slowly than other methods but provides a longer lasting freedom from cravings.

Nasal and Oral Nicotine Sprays

If none of the other methods appeal to you, a spray might be a good option. All you do with these is spray up your nose, like a saline or hay fever spray, or at the back of your throat, like a sore throat spray. Relief from nicotine cravings is reported to be close to immediate.

Bupropion

This medication does not contain nicotine, and it works by changing the way your brain and body reacts to the effects of nicotine. Basically, it affects the part of your brain that derives pleasure from smoking. Typically, you take this medication for a couple of weeks before your chosen quit date, and then continue taking it for about three months. During this time, the pleasure receptors in your brain will derive no pleasure from smoking, and will manage your cravings. Talk to your doctor if this option sounds appealing to you.

Varenicline

Like Bupropion, you start taking Varenicline up to two weeks before your chosen quit date, and continue taking it for about three months. During this time, your brain will react differently to the chemical contained in cigarette smoke. Many people reported quitting sooner than their quit date because they thought that the cigarettes tasted differently or made them feel nauseous, which put them off to smoking entirely. Talk to your doctor if this option sounds appealing to you.

Chapter 6: Therapeutic Techniques

Over the years, many smokers have opted to use therapeutic techniques to help with their smoking cessation efforts. Some of these techniques have higher success rates than others, and it is important to remember that what might work for someone else might not work for you. Some of these techniques will require you to find a practitioner, while other techniques are easy to learn and can be used at home or work.

Tai-Chi

In several studies, practicing Tai-Chi for one hour per day can drastically improve your chances of quitting smoking successfully. Tai-Chi gives you the relaxation that is typically reported by smokers after having a cigarette. Coupled with the fact that you are focused on your breathing and body, Tai-Chi makes you more conscious of the damage you are doing, and already have done, to your body. To check out a very cool Tai-Chi YouTube video by BodyWisdomTV click this link: Tai Chi for Beginners with Chris Pei.

Hypnosis

Hypnosis boasts upward of a forty percent success rate in helping people to quit smoking successfully. A recent study suggested that this method is likely to be more useful to men than women, however it also suggested that the success of hypnosis as a smoking cessation therapy is highly dependent on the suggestibility of the client and the skill of the hypnosis practitioner. You can also try hypnosis at home using one of the quit smoking sound tracks from HypnosisDownlods. Just download and then listen to it on your headphones once every day for several weeks while just sitting in a relaxing position or lying down in bed.

Acupuncture

Acupuncture practitioners and clients suggest that using acupuncture as a smoking cessation method improves your chances of quitting smoking successfully by up to thirty percent. Practitioners typically recommend a course of six to eight treatments with the first session taking place within seventy-two hours of quitting smoking. It is claimed that acupuncture increases serotonin levels in your brain, which counterbalances the serotonin reduction you will experience as you quit smoking.

Hand and Ear Massage

Maintaining serotonin levels can be an important part of managing nicotine cravings and quitting smoking successfully. A simple two minute massage of the ears is enough to increase serotonin levels in the brain, and a short self hand massage is enough to distract most anyone from lighting up a cigarette.

Mindful Meditation

Practicing mindful meditation for at least forty-five minutes every day can increase your chances of successfully quitting smoking by in excess of fifty percent.   Much like Tai-Chi, mindful meditation focuses heavily on breathing and body awareness, thus highlighting the damage you have done to your body by smoking. This awareness helps you to build an aversion to smoking. To see a great example of mindful meditation here is a great YouTube link. Mindful Meditation YouTube Link.

The first few weeks are the most important to quit smoking. Get through the first two weeks, and it will get easier and easier with each passing day. Utilize friends, family, and every strategy you read in this book to tough it out and get past the first two weeks. After that, it is much easier. This may mean not going out with friends who smoke, avoiding situations that you know will set you off, and actively visualizing yourself smoke free and utilizing all your resources for success in this endeavor!

The big tobacco companies have poured millions of dollars into designing the most addictive cigarettes that have ever been known to man. You are going to have to fight to be smoke free! Heaven knows it is a noble and worthy fight, and probably one of the top five things you can do in your entire life to be more successful. So don't give in! Do whatever it takes to keep yourself smoke free for life!

If you want to try and reduce some of the damage smoking may have done to you, be sure to check out my Anti-Aging book. Thank you and good luck!

Conclusion

I hope this book was able to help you to quit smoking. Only time will tell if your efforts will last, but you now know many methods now that will help you cope with future cravings and beat your nicotine addiction into the dirt once and for all.

The next step is to prepare yourself mentally and physically to be smoke free for good! Use the preparation techniques discussed in Chapter One to give yourself the best chances of quitting successfully. Millions of people every year quit smoking and live a healthier, happier, and wealthier life as a result. You can be one of them! It's your time now! Make a plan and follow through!

Finally, if you discovered at least one thing that has helped you or that you think would be beneficial to someone else, be sure to take a few seconds to easily post a quick positive review. As an author, your positive feedback is desperately needed. Your highly valuable five star reviews are like a river of golden joy flowing through a sunny forest of mighty trees and beautiful flowers! *To do your good deed in making the world a better place by helping others with your valuable insight, just leave a nice review.*

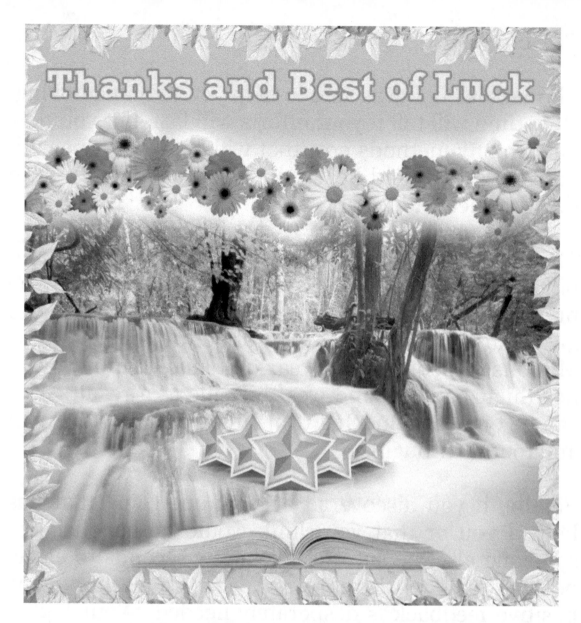

My Other Books and Audio Books
www.AcesEbooks.com

Health Books

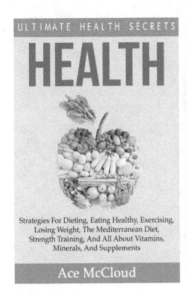

ULTIMATE HEALTH SECRETS

HEALTH

Strategies For Dieting, Eating Healthy, Exercising, Losing Weight, The Mediterranean Diet, Strength Training, And All About Vitamins, Minerals, And Supplements

Ace McCloud

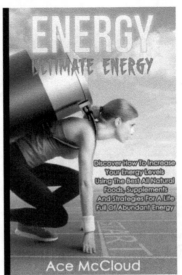

ENERGY
ULTIMATE ENERGY

Discover How To Increase Your Energy Levels Using The Best All Natural Foods, Supplements And Strategies For A Life Full Of Abundant Energy

Ace McCloud

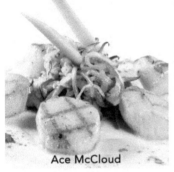

RECIPE BOOK

The Best Food Recipes That Are Delicious, Healthy, Great For Energy And Easy To Make

Ace McCloud

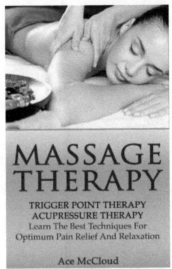

MASSAGE THERAPY

TRIGGER POINT THERAPY
ACUPRESSURE THERAPY
Learn The Best Techniques For Optimum Pain Relief And Relaxation

Ace McCloud

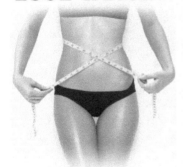

LOSE WEIGHT

THE TOP 100 BEST WAYS TO LOSE WEIGHT QUICKLY AND HEALTHILY

Ace McCloud

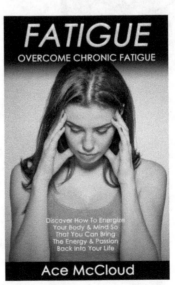

FATIGUE
OVERCOME CHRONIC FATIGUE

Discover How To Energize Your Body & Mind So That You Can Bring The Energy & Passion Back Into Your Life

Ace McCloud

Peak Performance Books

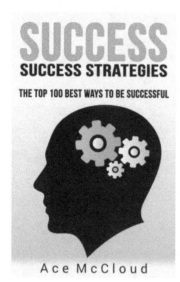

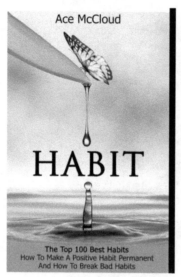

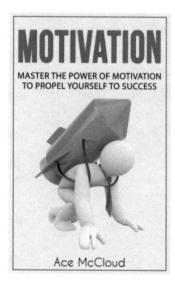

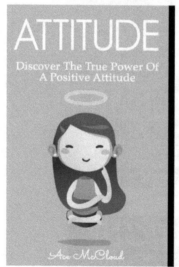

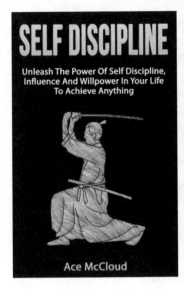

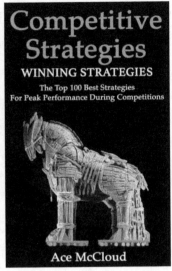

Be sure to check out my audio books as well!

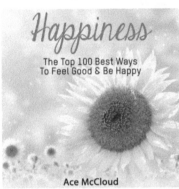

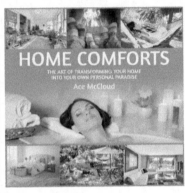

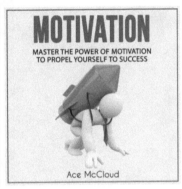

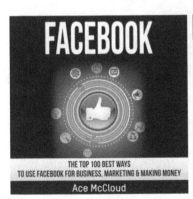

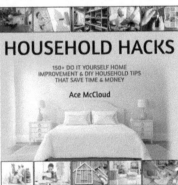

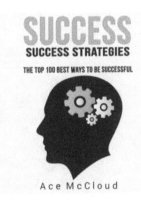

Check out my website at: www.AcesEbooks.com for a complete list of all of my books and high quality audio books. I enjoy bringing you the best knowledge in the world and wish you the best in using this information to make your journey through life better and more enjoyable! **Best of luck to you!**